Natural Health-Simplified

Your Personal Guide To Being Vital Again!

By

Dr. Heather Taylor-Hewett, N.D., C.H.P., C.C.H.

authorHOUSE®

AuthorHouse™
1663 Liberty Drive
Bloomington, IN 47403
www.authorhouse.com
Phone: 1 (800) 839-8640

Published by AuthorHouse 07/15/2017

ISBN: 978-1-4208-2540-4 (sc)
ISBN: 978-1-4634-8303-6 (e)

Print information available on the last page.

This book is printed on acid-free paper.

DEDICATION

I dedicate this book to my God Jehovah; my husband, Matt; and two sons, Jordan and Chandler, my parents, and grandmother. Without all of everyone's love and support, I would not have been able to accomplish my goals. Thanks also to Donna Faye, Inc., who has been supportive and helpful all the years I've known her.

TABLE OF CONTENTS

DEDICATION v

FOREWORD ix

CHAPTER ONE. GETTING STARTED-
ELIMINATING CONFUSION OF WHAT THE
NATURAL HEALTH LIFESTYLE IS ABOUT............. 1

    What Natural Health Is Not! 2

    Where Do I Begin Immediately? 3

CHAPTER TWO. "LET FOOD BE THY MEDICINE
AND MEDICINE BE THY FOOD"............................. 5

    What Do We Eat? 6

    My Recommendations For Your Children's
    Diet: 9

    Eliminate: 12

    What To Incorporate: 17

    Note Important Considerations For Optimal
    Health And Weight Loss: 18

CHAPTER THREE. HERBS - GOD'S MEDICINE
CABINET 24

    What exactly is an herb? 27

    The following herbs that should be in your
    medicine cabinet: 29

CHAPTER FOUR. HOMEOPATHY
INTERPRETED 33

    How it's prepared: 33

    Who it benefits: 34

CHAPTER FIVE. SUPPLEMENTS- ESSENTIAL
FOR LIFE: 35

    What do I take? 36

Explanations of recommendations: 36

CHAPTER SIX. ESSENTIAL OILS- THE LIFE
BLOOD OF PLANTS 38

How do you profit from using pure therapeutic
grade essential oils? 39

What is frequency and how does it coincide with
essential oils? 41

How do pure therapeutic grade essential oils
affect the brain? 41

CHAPTER SEVEN. COLON HYDROTHERAPY AND
LIVER DETOXIFICATION: 46

Why should I cleanse my body? 47

How do I get started? 48

Why is cleaning my liver so important to optimal
health? 50

Liver Stressors We Can Avoid: 51

How often should these cleanses be done? 52

CHAPTER EIGHT. POISONS THAT WILL
SABOTAGE ANYONE'S HEALTH AND WELL
BEING 53

REFERENCES: 65

FOREWORD

My dream has been to write a published book since I was a child. I imagined I would be a fictional writer. I never thought I would be inspired to write about self responsibility and self- healing. I had been duped into believing what medical science wants us to believe, that there was nothing you can do to reverse any type of illness you have been diagnosed with, and that you are an identifiable slave by it. I hope my journey will help encourage, motivate, and facilitate, your journey to unlock your body's unique ability to heal itself , be it illness of the mind or body.

CHAPTER ONE.
GETTING STARTED- ELIMINATING CONFUSION OF WHAT THE NATURAL HEALTH LIFESTYLE IS ABOUT

First of all, Natural health is a way of life. It's something that you emulate from the inside out. It's a way of life that becomes a blessing not a burden. Anything worth while in the beginning may be hard, but after modifications have been made, you wish you had done it sooner. Immediately you begin to feel alive again. You have more energy. Depression lifts and brain fogginess disappears. Natural health is a journey of self awareness. You become your body's friend again, not its enemy. You feel at peace mentally, emotionally, physically, and most important, spiritually. Natural health requires total body and mind adherence. For something new to truly work, it takes time and patience with yourself. So pace yourself and enjoy. Learn to listen to your body. Take one day at a time!

What Natural Health Is Not!

It's not about making 180 degree changes overnight. It's too costly financially, mentally, and physically. Your body gently needs changes. If anyone tells you to make changes overnight, run the other way. That's one of the reasons why fad diets only last a short time. In order for a new habit to work it has to be done a little at a time. Natural health is not a fad diet or a quick fix, it's for life! Living the lifestyle doesn't mean living like a hermit somewhere. You can't hide from pollution anywhere. What Natural Health does is teach you how to live healthfully anywhere you may be. This is not a new theory on health or a new or passing fad. Natural health has been around for centuries. Ayurvedic medicine is the world's oldest recorded healing system. It has been used for some 5,000 years. It has influenced other cultural medicines as well. The Chinese, Greeks, and Romans has originated their roots from Ayurvedic medicine. Our conventional medicine has only been around for 2-400 years at the most. What we call "Alternative medicine" here is standard practice in other countries. Natural health is here to stay. Millions each year are being spent on books, vitamins, and herbal remedies. Consumers are literally sick and tired of not getting better from the constant prescriptions and medications that are being written. We have new infections and viruses mutating constantly from the over prescribed antibiotics. It's time to take a look at what has been in front of us all along: natural remedies. Natural health is not about feeling helpless and falling victim to a diagnosed illness or disease, it's about taking responsibility for ourselves and what we put in our mouth. Natural health is not a quick cure all, but a gradual reversal of what imperfection has given us, as well as what we've done to ourselves.

Where Do I Begin Immediately?

I always recommend dietary changes first. The first thing I recommend to anyone who asks is to get some rich nutrition in your blood. I recommended a product called " SUPER NUTRITION." It's not a supplement ,it's an organic whole food. It's an actual meal replacement. It contains: spirulina, blue-green sea algae, chlorella-broken cell algae nettle leaf, purple dulse seaweed,wheatgrass, spinach leaf, alfalfa grass, barley grass, astragalus root, rose hips, orange peel, beet root, in a base of non active nutritional yeast. I have had patients come back to me and tell me they immediately noticed an energy increase. Who doesn't need that nowadays? You can get this product from(www.westernbotanicals.com.)   Then I recommend PLENTY OF PURE WATER! If one of your concerns in eating healthy is breaking your bank consider this: If you start drinking water and replace your coffee, soda, and commercial juice habits you'll save a money and unwanted empty calories! I would then suggest a new meal plan. After a healthy new meal plan is introduced and healthy new habits are started, then you can get into, detoxing, which I will cover later. I will educate you on herbs and their natural antibiotic actions, you'll learn about homeopathy, supplements, and poisons that are in your everyday food, water, and drinks. I hope that you will not let yourself be overwhelmed and remember anything worthwhile requires some

Dr. Heather Taylor-Hewett, N.D., C.H.P., C.C.H.

hardship, in the beginning. So keep an open mind. Remember, you only have your health to gain!

CHAPTER TWO.
"LET FOOD BE THY MEDICINE AND MEDICINE BE THY FOOD"

A quote by Hippocrates himself, (founding father of conventional medicine). What does this mean? Let's look at the typical American diet. The average American eats out several times a week. Everywhere you turn there's a fast food restaurant or a commercial about fast food. Why do Americans gluttonize themselves on this processed delicacy? It's about convenience, and because our bodies are confused. Nowadays, we work 40-50 hours a week, and we are rushing everywhere in our vehicles trying to get from point " a to point b." We are chronically stressed, which promotes hormonal imbalance, and eventually disease. Our nation leads the world in many diseases even though we have the "best medical care in the world." How can this contradiction be? Even the Surgeon General's Report on Nutrition and Health acknowledged, "What we eat may affect our risk for several of the leading causes of death for Americans; notably, the degenerative diseases such as: Atherosclerosis, Coronary Heart Disease, Stroke, Diabetes, and some types of Cancers.   With these disorders combined, they now account for more than two thirds of all deaths in the United States."   This concept of food is worth taking a look at.

What Do We Eat?

You may ask what do I eat? So much information out there, how do I know what's legitimately correct? My parents always told me to use common sense. Let's look at the food guide pyramid. This style of eating is, and has been used for years now. It's used in our school systems. The verdict: we have a nation full of obese children, with asthma and ear nose and throat infections. What is on their trays in school? An example taken from my younger sister's menu: hamburger with a white bun; sugary applesauce; white, or even worse ,chocolate milk; and a mixed vegetable that tastes like its been freezer- burned. How tantalizing and healthy! Yeah, right! Once a week they get fast food brought in from a local restaurant, as if they don't get enough of that already. No wonder our test scores are the worst in the nation, POOR NUTRITION! What do we do to either cut costs or try to give them a healthier lunch? We send them with " Lunchables", which is as processed as twinkies. As parents it is our responsibility to teach our children the correct way to nourish their bodies. Do I mean let them only eat flatbreads and raw brocolli? No, we want this new eating program to stick indefinitely. We start out slow, and do what I call tweeking the diet little by little. Get the children actively involved in planning school lunches and dinners. Let them have 1 junk food day a week. I'll give some examples: instead of white bread introduce whole grain bread, then eventually introduce sprouted grains which are the best, because its flourless. It contains about 5 grams of fiber per slice and is a moderate glycemic index food which we'll get to later. Cow's milk can be replaced with rice or goat's milk. Goat's milk is the closest to human milk and contains antibodies. Cow's milk contains allergy producing casein that is a protein that human's can't digest. It should only be consumed in it's raw form. The body's immune system reacts to the casein as if it were an invader and produces a lot of excessive mucous to try and rid the body of it. Therefore, we have a lot of children struggling with asthma and ear nose and throat infections. As you age, the process only gets worse. Cow's milk isn't the single cause of asthma and other illnesses like it, but it is a huge contributing factor. As far as the hamburger, only buy free range, grass fed, organic meats. They are free of pesticides, hormones and antibiotics. Pesticides contribute to many forms of cancers. Hormones are ingested and we have young girls starting their menstrual cycles too early and contributing to other imbalances in the body as well. Antibiotics weaken the immune system. Who wants that when we're struggling already? How about unsweetened applesauce? Or try another snack from the health food store. I'm tired of hearing, "The health food stores are so much more expensive than shopping at the big wharehouse stores." Guess what you spend a lot more on the non- healthy food than you realize. If you don't believe me, sit down and write out a list of what you spend a week on junk processed foods. Don't forget to add to the list, food eaten out. When I first calculated how much I spent on non healthy food , I was amazed. When you eat healthfully you don't eat as much, or as often. Your blood sugar stabilizes and your body is being properly nourished. You begin to lose the taste for junk food. Your children will only eat what is in your house. If you establish the precedent, they will follow. Implement the junk food day, so they won't feel deprived. It's worked for me. Think about how much time and money you'll save by not having to take off work and time lost sitting in their office waiting. My kids went from eating and drinking at every meal and snack some type of sugary food or drink..Remember, just because something is labeled organic doesn't mean 100% healthy. Some organic foods are loaded with sugar of some form. READ YOUR LABELS! If it lists too many ingredients, it's too processed. Remember adequate nutrition will yield a healthy body. What good ,is a juice that's organic with supplemental vitamins if it has 30 or more grams of sugar a serving. Fruit juices that sit on the shelves, are loaded with mold also. How important is low sugar intake? Remember this rule of thumb 40 or more grams of sugar slows the immune system by 70%. As you know, our immune systems protect us from a great deal of microbes as well as other harmful bacteria and viruses we come in contact with everyday. All of our children's favorite food and drinks are loaded with it. Just substitute their drink with water or fruit herbal teas or fresh squeezed juice. Does that mean substitute with artificial sweeteners? No! They are a bigger menace. For one, they can cause brain damage. Many studies have proven this. They're classified as neurotoxins. Recommended reading on just how much extensive damage can be done is the book entitled "EXCITOTOXINS THE TASTE THAT KILLS" by Russell L. Blaylock. The author is a board certified neurosurgeon. This book will blow you away. Another book for reading, is "FAST FOOD NATION " by Eric Schlosser. This a comprehensive look at the dangers of eating out. It will make you think twice about eating meat that is not organic.

My Recommendations For Your Children's Diet:

- 25- 40% of the diet should consist of protein (preferably animal sources since plant proteins are not complete proteins)

- low glycemic index organic fruits and vegetables unlimited, High glycemic index fruits and vegetables limit.

- whole grains and pastas (gluten free if allergic to wheat) limit the amount of grains consumed.

- plenty of distilled, artesian, or reverse osmosis water

- dairy should only be organic rice or organic goat's milk

- LIMIT REFINED SUGAR!

Implement these ideas and immediately you'll notice less allergic reactions. Proper supplementation is important too. An important point to remember it's not what you take it's what you absorb. I highly recommend Thorne supplements. They prepare only "hypoallergenic"-definition: non allergy producing. Thorne is the only company which uses the purest ingredients available. Their products contain no lubricants made of indigestible ingredients which prevent you from absorbing the active nutrients.

Yes, they are a little spendy, but you can be sure you're getting your money's worth because you're assimilating all the nutrients. Any other product you may be wasting your money.

I would definitely recommend you reading: "The No Grain Diet" by Dr. Mercola and "The Metabolic Typing Diet" by William Wolcott and Trish Fahey. If you're serious about feeling and looking your best, these books will help you get there. It doesn't advocate any crash dieting or counting calories or fat grams. They help you to appreciate that one meal plan doesn't fit everyone. It lifts the shroud of confusion of looking and feeling your best. Our bodies are designed to assimilate foods from whole and appropiate sources. Case and point; the vehicles we drive require a certain type of fuel with a specific octane level to run efficiently and to avoid premature breakdown. Likewise, our body engines require a specific fuel to run efficiently. What would happen if you used a lower octane for a car that requires a high octane gas? Sure you may get away with it for a while but problems would start to occur prematurely. Why? the vehicle was <u>designed </u>to take a specific type of gas. Our bodies function similiarly. If we abuse our bodies by putting processed fuel in our bodies, we will not only breakdown faster but we will soon have to contend with illnesses we didn't have to get. Some of us suffer from allergies, which is your body telling you it has toxic overload and your immune system is on high alert because your liver can't deal with the overload of chemicals from the environment and the food and drink were consuming.

I will give a brief summary of each book: "The Metabolic Typing Diet" asserts that one man's medicine is another man's poison. We are categorized into three basic types: slow oxidizers, fast oxidizers, and mixed oxidizers. It even gives you a test to see where you would fall individually as a unique person. Metabolic typing is the culmination of seventy years of pioneering efforts and interrelated discoveries by a whole series of remarkable medical researchers, including physicians, biochemists, physiologists, clinical nutritionists, dentists, and psychologists. The authors give some criteria that separates this type of eating from the rest by these disciplines: 1. Metabolic typing is applicable to chronic health disorders 2. Metabolic typing moves beyond symptom -oriented medicine. 3. Metabolic typing produces reliable, predictable clinical results. 4. Metabolic typing offers a highly integrated approach to building health. 5. Metabolic typing relies on the body's innate intelligence. 6. Metabolic typing represents a logical new paradigm shift. This book will answer a lot of unanswered questions. It's definitely worth looking into.

"The No Grain Diet" proves how the obesity epidemic is linked to grain consumption, and not, fat consumption. Dr. Mercola helps you see why most diets fail, and how you can conquer carbohydrate addiction physically, mentally, and emotionally. Which I've never seen anyone address before. These books are definitely a must read. So if you're serious about getting the most out of what you consume and feeling vital again, please read and implement the suggested meal plans for your type.

Important considerations for optimal health;

First, what to eliminate! These culprits are undesirables that need to be removed right away, because they are causitive factors for brain damage and serious diseases:

Eliminate:

EXCITOTOXINS (DEFINITION: A substance added to foods and beverages that literally stimulates neurons in your brain to death, causing brain damage of varying degrees. It's best known as MSG (monosodiumglutamate).

Additives that always contain MSG:

Monosodium Glutamate

Hydrolyzed Vegetable Protein

Hydrolyzed Protein

Hydrolyzed Plant Protein

Plant Protein Extract

Sodium Caseinate

Calcium Caseinate

Yeast Extract

Texturized Protein

Autolyzed Yeast

Hydrolyzed Oat Flour

Additives that frequently contain MSG:

Malt Extract

Malt Flavoring

Bouillon

Broth

Stock

Flavoring

Natural Flavoring

Natural Beef or Chicken Flavoring

Seasoning

Spices

Additives that may contain MSG or excitoxins:

Carrageenan

Enzymes

Soy Protein Concentrate

Soy Protein Isolate

Whey Protein Concentrate

Protein enzymes of various sources can release excitoxin amino acids.

Dr. Heather Taylor-Hewett, N.D., C.H.P., C.C.H.

OTHER EXCITOXINS:

Nutrasweet

Aspartic acid

Aspartame

Cysteine

Aspartate

Glutamate

NOTE: IN LIQUID FORM, EXCITOXINS CAUSE MORE DAMAGE! DIET DRINKS CONTAIN ARTIFICIAL SWEETNERS THAT ARE CLASSIFIED AS EXCITOXINS.

EXCITOXINS have been implicated in being a contributing factor to these diseases: diabetes, obesity, seizures, headaches, brain injury, fetal brain damage, (especially babies and toddlers) ALS, Anoxia, Hypoglycemia, Brain Tumors, A.D.D., A.D.H.D., Depression, Manic Depression, Mood Disorders, Chronic Fatigue, Parkinson's Disease, Alzheimers, Stroke and Ischemia.

They are in most processed foods. Please note just because a label or restaurant says "no MSG" doesn't mean this is so. Check your labels for ingredients! MSG is hidden in the above mentioned additives. As you're reading this now new additives are being formed to fool the public because it is cheap and a huge profit maker. Lobbying has been done since the 1980's by top neuroscientists for these additives to be outlawed, but the FDA has turned their head and looked the other way, They have too much to lose in regards to profit!

<u>OTHER FOOD AND DRINK TO ELIMINATE</u>:

Store bought fruit juices (high in sugar and mold)

All sodas (high in sugar and leaches phosphorus from your bones)

coffee (caffeine is lethal and has more uric acid than a cup of your urine)

white refined foods (breads, rice)

Refined and artificial sugar (contributes to insulin resistance, causing diabetes, obesity, heart disease)

Margarine and vegetable spreads (contain trans fatty acids, the evil fat that cause heart disease)

Corn sweetners (spikes high insulin levels)

Sushi (contains high levels of parasites)

Fried foods (cause health problems and carcinogenic)

Canned foods (contains high levels of mercury)

Alcohol (loaded with chemicals and insulin spiker, red European wine is ok because it doesn't contain nitrates)

Hydrogenated oils (they are trans fats)

Smoking (causes cancer and pollutes the environment, second hand smoke kills!)

Dr. Heather Taylor-Hewett, N.D., C.H.P., C.C.H.

Recreational and Pharmaceutical drugs (both damage liver and are both Excitoxins)

Birth Control Pill or any other synthetic hormone replacement (causes fibroids and other tumors, r depression, weight gain, and other illnesses, because you're ingesting PREGNANT HORSE URINE!)

Vegetable cooking oils: corn, safflower, sunflower, canola, sesame, soybean, and other monounsaturated oils. (these oils are trans fats and are toxic when used at high temperatures)

Simple carbs(spikes high insulin levels)

Why is control of your insulin levels so important? If not kept under control, illness will take hold. These high ranking disease all stem from out- of -control insulin levels: heart disease, diabetes, high blood pressure, high cholesterol, and obesity which kills 500,000 people a year!

The fact is any food or drink high in carbohydrates from grains or sugar cause a rapid spike in your blood glucose (sugar). Your pancreas, because of this surge of sugar, will compensate by secreting the hormone insulin into the bloodstream, which then lowers your blood sugar causing hypoglycemia. Insulin is actually a storage hormone. It stands to reason that too much insulin, equals more fat storage! High insulin levels lower two other important hormones :glucagon and growth hormone- that are responsible for burning fat and sugar and promoting muscle development. Insulin causes a false signal of feeling hungry. That is why soon after a high carbohydrate or starchy meal you feel hungry again and usually for sweets! Continue in this pattern and you'll ride a roller coaster of emotions and you will gain weight and be depressed, fatigued, and sick.

The more you cut out grains and starchy fruit and vegetables the more alert, lean, healthy, youthful, and mentally and emotionally stable you'll become.

What To Incorporate:

Plenty of organic vegetables (usually the darker the better)

Plenty of pure water (consume at least half of your body weight in ounces, drink distilled or ionized or ozonated water

Organic fruits that are low in starch (high starch fruits have a high impact on blood glucose levels)

Super nutrition green drink (high in vitamins, minerals, and enzymes.)

Coconut oil (full of nutrition, helps fight many diseases and illnesses, helps weight loss, provides energy, regulates blood sugar, antimicrobial, antifungal properties, keeps skin and hair young and healthy when used internally and externally) Be careful of the type you buy. Make sure of these important factors: it must be certified organic, USDA standards, no refining, no chemicals added, no bleaching, no deodorization, no hydrogenation, non- GMO, from traditional palms- no hybrid varieties, from fresh coconuts, not the dried "copra" used in most coconut oils, low level heated only so it does not damage nutrients. Check out *Mercola.com* for great tasting coconut oil and organic, grass fed, meats.

Proper supplementation (will discuss in later chapter)

Supplemental enzymes (helps with digestion of cooked food)

Regular excercise

Probiotics (friendly bacteria)

Regular colon, liver, kidney, anti-parasite detox programs (only under practioner supervision)

Green tea and Yerba mate herbal teas (make sure tea is organic and not smoked) *Ecoteas.com* has great quality teas at an awesome value. Benefits of teas include: lowers cholesterol; blood pressure; and prevents platelet aggregation; prevents heart disease; inhibits initiation, promotion, and progression of cancer; bolsters immunity and has anti-microbial properties. It is an inhibitor of Pneumonia; Whooping Cough; dental bacteria; and viral infections; aids in the proper function of the liver, which helps detoxify the body; promotes healthy cognitive functions- great for depression and brain fogginess; packed with vitamins; minerals; and antioxidants. Green tea contains a moderate amount of caffeine (not as much as coffee). Yerba mate contains a gentler stimulant called " mateine" which is a cousin of caffeine. These are great alternatives to coffee!

Note Important Considerations For Optimal Health And Weight Loss:

Limit your consumption of grains and sugar. Grains should only be eaten as a whole grain, and best of all sprouted. Sprouted grains are 100% flourless and contains all essential amino acids; rich in protein, vitamins, minerals, and natural fiber with no added fat. Stay away from corn and corn products; it is an insulin spiker and is fed to livestock to fatten them up. A diet high in corn products, (remember many processed foods contain some type of corn), has shown to negatively impact one's health. There's been evidence of anemia, dental cavities, osteoarthritis, infections, and other health issues because of corn's high sugar content. Corn derivatives are as follows: corn syrup, fructose corn syrup, high fructose corn syrup, corn oil, cornmeal, cornstarch, dextrose, monosodium glutamate, xanthan gum, and maltodextrin. There are two more risks to consider besides the high sugar content of corn. Corn is only second to soybeans as the most genetically modified crop in the U.S. There have been no studies done on GMO foods and their negative impact on human health. Another risk factor is corn is one of the foods highest in **mycotoxins** (wheat and other grains as well) which are toxins from fungus that can lead to cancer, heart disease, diabetes, and a wide range of other illnesses.

SUGAR- wreaks havoc on your health. It can act as a cancer ravaging every healthy cell in your body. Do not underestimate its effects. It is a causitive factor in many conditions and illnesses such as:

overweight and obesity

immune system suppression

premature aging

cancer

Dr. Heather Taylor-Hewett, N.D., C.H.P., C.C.H.

decreased absorption of calcium and magnesium

chronic fatigue

heart disease

digestive illnesses

osteoporosis

yeast infections candida

depression

manic depression

dental caries and gum disease

high cortisol levels(the death hormone)

There are many other illnesses sugar has been implicated in. Heart disease is caused by too much arterial plaque build- up and the main culprit is sugar. It's sticky residue causes arterial damage and high cholesterol and is the culprit behind heart disease. Fats have received all the blame for heart disease, when in fact, since the onset of no-fat and low fat dieting, heart disease and diabetes have reached epic proportions. Clearly fat isn't the only villain here.

Soybeans are popular right now and are touted for being a healthy alternative to many foods. They aren't a healthy choice. I bet right now your mouth is dropping; yes, soy is not a healthy option. Many people actually have an intolerance or allergy to soy. Soybeans are used in various processed foods. Asians are by far a healthier people and do use soy in their diet you may say, but they use only fermented soy such as natto, amakaze, miso, and tempeh. When used in its fermented form, any negative effects are negated. Consider these points about soybeans:

- soybeans are high in natural toxins, also known as "antinutrients". This would include a large quantity of inhibitors that deter the enzymes needed for protein digestion. The result is extensive gastric distress and chronic defiencies in amino acid uptake, which can result in pancreatic impairment and cancer.

- they contain hemaglutamin, which cause red blood cells to clump together. Soybeans also have growth depressant factors.

- contains gotrogens, which leads to thyroid depression

- most soybeans are genetically modified, and they contain on of the highest levels of pesticide contamination of all foods.

- soybeans are high in phytates, which prevent absorption of minerals including calcium, magnesium, iron, and zinc.

- soybeans are taken through an acid washing in aluminum tanks in an effort to remove antinutrients and are found to have a heavy aluminum content.

- Many soy foods have toxic levels of manganese.

- soybeans increase high estrogen levels

Coconut oil is the healthiest oil you can consume. What is she talking about you may ask?

Dr. Heather Taylor-Hewett, N.D., C.H.P., C.C.H.

The media told us a decade ago that coconut oil was high in fat and will lead to heart disease. I remember that broadcast well. It was centered around movie popcorn. They found that movie popcorn was popped in coconut oil. After the bad press the movie theaters changed the oil to vegetable oils. What a mistake, since vegetable oils are high in omega 6 oils that cause an imbalance in our bodies. An imbalance left unchecked leads to disease. Vegetable oils such as canola, safflower, sunflower, and corn lead to hypothyroidism and a lowered metabolic rate. Coconuts are high in saturated fat but contrary to popular belief are necessary for nutrition. There are different types of saturated fat. Coconut oil is a medium chained fatty acid and digested more easily and utilized by the body differently. Other fats are stored in the body's cells where as coconut oil's fat is sent directly to your liver to be converted as energy. The oil in coconuts heat up your metabolic furnace. Coconuts are high in protein and low in carbs. They are good sources of folic acid, all B vitamins, and minerals including calcium, magnesium, and potassium. Olive oil is a good oil to use as well. Coconut's health benefits far exceed olive oils. Since olive oil is a monounsaturated fat it is more susceptible to oxidative damage when used in cooking. When buying coconut oil look for these standards:[certified organic, USDA standards]

no refining

no chemical added

no bleaching

no deodorization

no hydrogenation

non GMO

from traditional palms only no hybrid varieties

from fresh coconuts not the dried "copria" used in most coconut oils

low level heated only so nutrients aren't damaged

Ask yourself this question each time you pick up an undesirable thing to eat : "Is this worth all the negative effects on my health?" Answer honestly. If you give in, could it be emotional eating then? What need does this food offer me? Can I busy myself with other things? Remember it's up to you to be diligent in your endeavor for optimal health for you. I didn't say perfect health, I said optimal health for you!

CHAPTER THREE.
HERBS - GOD'S MEDICINE CABINET

There is much confusion about herbs these days. We hear a lot of negative reports from the media as well as from misinformed magazine publications. Herbs are being labeled as dangerous and are ripped of the shelves. There is a saying, " people fear what they fully don't understand." Vitamin and supplement companies are all racing to get the latest and greatest herb product out there without fully taking the time and money to clearly understand the power and purpose behind herbs. They sloppily and mistakenly use standardized extracts instead of the whole herb. It's dangerous to use a part of an herb when the other part that has been left behind acts as a balancer so harsh side effects won't occur. A classic example is Ephedra or Mahaung . The standardized extract is normally used in products and not the whole leaf . When you add to that abuse of the herb by young teenagers and athletes looking for a quick energy fix, dehydration, and intense heat and humidity, you have a recipe for trouble. The government comes under fire for it and instead of investigating fully, they ban it. What about all the poisonous pharmaceutical drugs on the market? I was once told by a nurse in an emergency hospital, if someone really wanted to kill themselves they should overdose on Tylenol- that will stop your liver from functioning. To me, the moral of the story is if you overdose on most things you'll hurt yourself or worst yet kill yourself. So please, use herbs in moderation and use organic good quality herbs from a reputable company. I suggest using Western Botanicals . They're a company that stays true to what herbs and healing are all about. They have there own website www.westernbotanicals.com . I highly recommend seeing a Naturopathic Doctor or Holistic Health Practioner and avoid self- medicating.

How do herbs work? Herbs are so powerful they can easily replace our modern day antibiotics. Our pharmaceutical antibiotics are simple substances with only one chemical constitute to kill bacteria. They are successful in killing bacteria but they leave harmful toxins behind and kill all good bacteria as well; therefore, setting the body up for something even more lethal in the future. Another drawback to antibiotics is that the bacteria it was created to kill develops an immunity to it, thereby causing a stronger antibiotic to be used for other infections, and the vicious cycle continues. In contrast herbs are complex and possess many constitutes instead of just one so bacteria can't easily figure out how to counteract it. Therefore, an immunity can't be built against the herbs used. For example: yarrow, a powerful herbal antibiotic contains over 120 different compounds that have been discovered so far. When someone uses yarrow for an infection, they're actually taking in over

120 different medicines. All of these medicines coexist in balance, and enhance, potentiate, and mitigate each other's effects inside the body. Why won't the pharmaceutical companies use these herbs ? They actually do use some herbs, but again, they don't use the <u>entire</u> herb, use only part of it, and then mix it with other man- made substances. In this way they can patent their creation and make billions of dollars off it. They can't patent herbs in its whole form, and the profit and markup just isn't there like it is for their chemical creations. I will list the top antibiotic herbs in alphabetical order;

ACACIA

ALOE

CRYPTOLEPSIS

ECHINACEA

EUCALYPTIS

GARLIC

GINGER

GOLDENSEAL

GRAPEFRUITSEED EXTRACT

HONEY

JUNIPER

LICORICE

SAGE

USNEA

WORMWOOD

These herbs have more than one or two uses. They can even be used for ailments, as well as problems such as depression.

An important point is that herbs have always been at the center of medicine, holistic or otherwise. Herbs are used today in about 25 percent of all prescription drugs. For the most part, though, modern medicine has ventured off the path of using pure herbs in the treatment of disease and other health disorders. Most, in part because of greed, and the other reason is because most people want a miracle quick- fix drug, instead of taking responsibility and patiently addressing the real cause of a malady. Another reason is that herbs cannot be patented and drug companies cannot hold the exclusive right to sell a specific herb. The collection and preparation of herbal medicine cannot be as easily controlled as the manufacture of synthetic drugs making its profits less dependable. Despite negative publicity, herbal medicine is on the uprise again. Millions were spent last year on some type of herbal formula. The reasons are simple most people are fed up with harmful side effects of pharmaceutical drugs. If one has any doubt as to the role that herbs have played in medicine all one would have to do is look in the <u>United States Pharmacopoeia</u>.

What exactly is an herb?

The word " herb" is used in herbal medicine (also known as botanical medicine or in Europe as phytotherapy or phytomedicine), means a plant or plant part that is used to make medicine, food flavors (spices) or aromatic oils for soaps and fragrances. An herb can be a leaf, a stem, a flower, a seed, a root, a fruit, bark, or any other plant part and is used for its food flavoring, fragrant properties, and for its medicinal properties. Throughout history cultural knowledge of medicinal uses of herbs has been passed down from generation to generation to our day. Negative reporting from the media has indicated that many herbs don't work and people should avoid buying them. When you look into the actual reports again, standardized extracts, along with poor quality herbs, have been used in case studies. The quality of herb is just as important as the type of herb used. Herbs come in many forms, whole, teas, capsules and tablets, extracts and tinctures, in essential oils, salves, balms, and ointments. Tinctures are my favorite because they are the most potent form of it. They have the advantage of high concentration in low weight and space. They are quickly assimilated in the bloodstream. All of these forms have advantages to whatever you need them for.

What can herbs be used for? They have a wide range of uses starting with: minor ailments; digestive complaints, depression, skin rashes, cold and flu, menstrual complaints, insomnia, sunburn, diarrhea and constipation, and many others. Other conditions respond well to herbal medicine such as: peptic ulcers, heartburn, rheumatic and arthritic conditions, eczema and psoriasis, anxiety and nerve disorders, bronchitis, parasitic conditions, allergies and asthma, diabetes, and hypertension. These are just a few ailments that can be treated with herbal medicine. Literally, every ailment can be treated with herbal medicine. I myself treated many illnesses and ailments of my own over the years with great success. Please don't self diagnose and treat yourself without the guidance of a certified herbal medicine practioner or naturopathic doctor. Their knowledge and expertise can guide you to the right type of herbal medicine for you. Do not overlook herbs because of their seemingly simplisitc nature. Remember, we learned that herbs are not simple in constitution like pharmaceutical drugs are, they contain many compounds for healing. Don't under- estimate their power to heal.

The following herbs that should be in your medicine cabinet:

Aloe vera- great for sunburns and all other burns

Arnica flowers- use externally for soft tissue injuries, like dislocations, sprains cuts, wound healing, bruises, varicose ulcers. Dilute with oil.

Cayenne pepper fruit- use internally for the chill stage of a fever, debility and convalescence in old age, varicose veins, asthma, digestive problems, and heart attack. Use externally for sprains, unbroken chilblains, neuralgia, lumbago, and pleurisy.

Dandelion root- A good general tonic. Relieves stomach cramps, is a diuretic and helps chronic skin conditions, such as rashes, eczema, and acne. Brings relief to liver inflammation. Use internally for gall bladder, and urinary disorders, gallstones, jaundice, cirrhosis, dyspepsia with constipation, edema associated with high blood pressure and heart weakness, chronic joint and skin complaints, gout, eczema, and acne.

Ginger rhizome- Use internally for motion sickness, nausea, morning sickness, indigestion , colic, abdominal, chills, colds, coughs, influenza, and peripheral circulation problems. Use externally for rheumatism, lumbago, menstrual cramps, sprains, spasmodic pain.

Lobelia herb- Use internally for asthma, bronchitis, whooping cough, and pleurisy as a general nerve and muscle relaxant or to induce vomiting. Use externally for pleurisy, rheumatism, tennis elbow, whiplash injuries, boils, and ulcers.

Catnip- Use internally for feverish illnesses, insomnia, excitability, palpitations, nervous indigestion, diarrhea, stomach upsets, and colic.

Peppermint- Use for toothache, nausea, colic, gas, headache, insomnia, fevers and dysentary.

Mullein leaf- Soothing and calming. Great for breaking up mucous congestion. Use internally for coughs, whooping cough, bronchitis, laryngitis, tonsillitis, tracheitis, asthma, influenza, excess respiratory mucus, tuberculosis, urinary infections, nervous tension, and insomnia. Use externally for earaches, sores, wounds, boils, blisters, rheumatic pain, hemorrhoids, and chilblains. Use as a skin wash for soothing and easing pain.

Myrrh gum- Astringent, antiseptic, and antimicrobial. Mostly effective for sore throats, canker sores, gingivitis. For any mouth, gum, throat, or digestive problems. Will increase white blood cell count.

Nettle leaf- Use internally for allergies, anemia, hemorrhage. Use for fatigue or exhaustion. Good for liver, gallbladder, and spleen disorders, headaches anemia, blood disorders, colds/flu, allergies, excessive menstruation, hemorrhoids, arthritis, rheumatism, gout, and skin complaints (especially eczema). Use externally for arthritic pain, gout, sciatica, neuralgia, hemorrhoids, scalp and hair problems, burns, insect bites, and nosebleed.

White oat bark- Use internally to reduce inflammation, control diarrhea, chronic nosebleeds and hemorrhoids, bleeding gums, minor injuries, dermatitis, weeping eczema, ringworm, ulcers, and varicose veins.

Valerian- use internally for insomnia, hysteria, anxiety, cramps, migraines, indigestion of nervous origin, hypertension, and painful menstruation. Externally for eczema, ulcers, and minor injuries (especially splinters).

Yarrow- This a powerful healer and purifier. Use internally for feverish illnesses(especially colds, influenza, and measles), mucus, diarrhea, lack of appetite, gas, nose bleeds, general hemorrhage, muscular pain, stomach disorders or bleeding, dyspepsia/indigestion, rheumatism, arthritis, menstrual and menopausal complaints, colds/flu, skin infections, boils and pimples, hypertension, and to protect against thrombosis after stroke or heart attack.

Yellow dock root- Use internally for chronic skin diseases, jaundice, constipation (especially associated with skin eruptions acne) liver disorders, and anemia.

You will find there will be no side effects if not abused, and bacteria will not be able to resist the many compounds they come in contact with. They have a long shelf life and won't break the bank like antibiotics

Dr. Heather Taylor-Hewett, N.D., C.H.P., C.C.H.

and other pharmaceutical drugs will. Please see an herbalist or natural health care professional.

CHAPTER FOUR.
HOMEOPATHY INTERPRETED

Homeopathy is a non toxic system of medicine that millions of people use with much success. They are usually dilutions of substances found in nature like; plants, minerals, and animals. It is based on the "like for like" principle, or law of similiars. It actually has a 180 year history of use. One popular remedy you may have seen in the stores is *"oscillococcinum"*. It's origin is from France and is growing in popularity here for the ease of cold symptoms. Homeopathy was founded by German physician, Samuel Hahneman. He's been known for his work in pharmacology, hygiene, public health, industrial toxicology, and psychiatry. He feels the more dilute the remedy the greater its potency.

How it's prepared:

It's prepared through a process of diluting with pure water or alcohol and succussing (vigorously shaking). They can be made by being diluted to such an extent that literally no molecules of the original substance remain in the remedy. The explanation actually lies in the realm of quantum physics and the emerging field of energy medicine.

Who it benefits:

Anyone with any condition will benefit from emotional and mental disorders to diabetes to cancer. There has been many documented cases of people who have benefitted from homeopathy. It's a great and better alternative to pharmaceutical poisons out there. Please consider the book "Homeopathy Made Simple" by Dr. R. Donald Papen. It has a fully complete, easy to read comprehensive chart on homeopathic remedies on what and how to use them.

CHAPTER FIVE.
SUPPLEMENTS- ESSENTIAL
FOR LIFE:

This is a hotly debatable topic. Some health care professionals will disagree with my adherence of the use of supplements. The claim has been made that if you have a "perfect diet" of organic fresh fruit and vegetables, you don't need supplemention. I say hogwash because of environmental pollution and the ground so devoid of adequate minerals. How can anyone get an adequate supply of the needed vitamins and minerals? Add to that, daily stress and the constant baragement of parasites, and unwanted bacterial and viral invaders. Let's face it, we need positive reinforcements that are called supplements. I do not mean supplement without healthful eating. If you do that you're probably not assimilating the proper nutrients. I recommend a diet of plenty of fresh organic fruits and vegetables, plenty of juicing, some protein, and limited grains. Detoxification is essential for assimilation of nutrients as well. If you have a rancid colon you will not assimilate nutrients properly!

Dr. Heather Taylor-Hewett, N.D., C.H.P., C.C.H.

Remember, "**supplememt**" means: something added to make up for a lack or deficiency. That's all, these are not a substitute for a proper diet.

What do I take?

Again, I recommend Super Nutrition as mentioned in the earlier chapter on food. A good multivitamin for your specific needs. A good omega 3 formula, probiotics, enzymes, and a Colon Cleanse formula. This is a good foundational approach for anyone seeking optimal health. I highly recommend <u>Thorne</u> products. They can be found at <u>www.thorne.com.</u> Again, I plead with you to see a naturopathic doctor that will do a hair mineral analysis to see what you actually need so you will help support your body, not work against it. A good point to keep in mind- it's not only <u>what</u> you put in your mouth but what you <u>assimilate</u>.

Supplementation is also important because when the body is without adequate supplies of vitamins, minerals, and amino acids, complications arise in the body's delicate balance of precision. If left unchecked disease and illness sets in.

Explanations of recommendations:

• A good multivitamin and mineral supplement will be a complete comprehensive formula as I previously stated you can get from Thorne.

• omega 3 formula should consist of Epa and Dha (Omega 3 is essential for healthy brain function for children and adults.)

- probiotics are friendly bacteria that the body needs for a healthy immune system and healthy intestines. Use a formula that has lactobacillous spores in it so it will colonize your colon, not just pass through your intestines.

- supplemental enzymes are important for eating any food that is not raw. Raw foods contain their own enzymes to digest themselves. Enzymes in supplemental form will help break down foods during digestion so you won't have to waste your body's enzymes.

- Colon Cleanse is necessary to keep the intestinal tract free of harmful candida and parasites. It aids in the removal of fecal matter. Do not buy a harsh laxative. I recommend Western Botanicals Colon Cleanse products. It is merely an herbal aid, not a harsh chemical stimulant.

Implement these supplements with a healthful eating plan and exercise and you'll be well on your way to feeling vital!

CHAPTER SIX.
ESSENTIAL OILS- THE LIFE BLOOD OF PLANTS

This is my second favorite chapter. After cleansing and detoxification is done, essential oils are highly recommended by many avid users of the oils. I can attest to this they have really changed my life.

When were they first founded and used for healing? Essential oils were mankind's first medicine. Proof of that is clearly seen in ancient writings such as Chinese manuscripts, Egyptian hieroglyphics, and the Bible, which is the most ancient book of all. There are over 188 references to essential oils in the Bible. God's chosen people at the time were to use these oils for very specific purposes in their worship to Him.

What are clean, pure, therapeutic grade essential oils, and why is it necessary for oils to be unadulterated? First essential oils are the volatile liquids that are distilled from plants (including their respective parts, such as : seed, bark, leaves, roots, flowers, fruit, and stems, etc). The oil's chemical constitutes determine their purity and therapeutic value. These delicate constitutes can be affected by a number of factors including: the parts of the plant from which the oil was produced, the soil, fertilizer (being organic or chemical) the geographical location, climate, altitude, the harvest methods and seasons, and the distillation process. Undoubtedly, there is a need for pure therapeutic- grade essential oils whether for personal use or for healthcare. Weak substitutes do not qualify or replace pure therapeutic grade oils. If you choose to use a cheap substitute you will not get the desired effect. I highly recommend **Young Living Essential Oils**. I haven't found anything that even compares. These oils are so pure you can take them internally. Anything that you use on your skin you should be able to ingest without harm. Everything that comes in contact with your skin will eventually turn up in your bloodstream. So think about that for a minute. Is saving a few bucks worth getting cancer?

How do you profit from using pure therapeutic grade essential oils?

1. Essential oils are the regenerating, oxygenating, and immune defense properties of plants (their life blood).

2. Essential oils are so small in molecular size they're transdermal; meaning ,they can quickly penetrate the tissues of the skin.

3. Essential oils are lipid soluble and are able to penetrate cell walls, even if they have hardened because of an oxygen deficiency. They can be metabolized by the body in 20 minutes.

4. Essential oils contain oxygen molecules which help to transport nutrients to human cells.

5. Essential oils are powerful antioxidants.

6. Essential oils are antibacterial, anti-fungal, anti-infectious, antimicrobial, anti-tumoral, anti-cancerous, anti-parasitic, anti-viral, and antiseptic.

7. Essential oils may detoxify the blood and cells in the body.

8. Essential oils containing sesquiterpenes have the ability to pass the blood brain barrier, which enables them to be effective in treating Parkinson's , Alzheimer's , Lou Gehrig's Disease and, multiple sclerosis.

9. Essential oils are aromatic. When they are diffused, they provide air purification by performing the following tasks: removing metallic particles and toxins form the air, they increase atmospheric, oxygen, they increase ozone and negative ions in the area which inhibits bacterial growth, they destroy odors from mold, cigarettes, and animals, and they fill the air with a fresh clean scent.

10. Essential oils help promote emotional, spiritual, and physical healing.

11. Essential oils have a bio-electrical frequency that is several times greater than the frequency of herbs, food, and even the human body. Clinical studies have shown that essential oils can quickly raise the frequency of the human body, restoring it to it's normal healthy level.

What is frequency and how does it coincide with essential oils?

First of all , frequency is a measurable rate of electrical energy that is constant between any two points. Everything has an electrical frequency. There is actually equipment that was invented to measure the bio frequency of humans and food. The human body has 62-68 MHZ. Processed/canned food has 0 MHZ, fresh produce has up to 15MHZ , fresh herbs, 20-27 MHZ, and essential oils has anywhere from 52-320 MHZ. Another reason I hate coffee, a test was done with two subjects- the first person was a 26 year old male, the second was a 24 year old male. They were measured first for a frequency of 66 MHZ. The first person held a cup of coffee, and his frequency dropped to 58 MHZ in 3 seconds. He then removed the coffee then inhaled an aroma of essential oils. Within 21 seconds, his frequency had returned to 66MHZ. The second person took a sip of coffee and his frequency dropped to 52 MHZ in the same 3 seconds. NO essential oils were administered during recovery time and it took 3 days for his frequency to return to the initial 66MHZ. Why is this important you ask ? Death begins at 25 MHZ, so let's say you have candida, like most people in America, and you drank coffee. Your frequency would drop to 41. Why is this serious? Well, cancer begins when you have a frequency of only 42MHZ. Essential oils are the missing link in today's modern world to optimal health.

How do pure therapeutic grade essential oils affect the brain?

It's important to first understand what the blood brain barrier is. It is the barrier membrane between the circulating blood and the brain that prevents certain damaging substances from reaching brain tissue and cerebrospinal fluid.

High levels of sesquiterpines , found in certain essential oils, help increase the amount oxygen in the limbic system of the brain in particular, around the pineal and pituitary glands. This oxygenating effect will lead to an increase in secretion of antibodies, endorphins, and neurotransmitters. The American Medical Association found and determined that if they could find an agent that would pass the blood brain barrier, they would be able to cure Alzheimer's, Lou Gehrig's , Parkinson's and Multiple Sclerosis.   Important to note that in June of 1994, it was documented by the Medical University of Berlin, Germany, and Vienna, Austria that sesquiterpines have the ability to go beyond the blood brain barrier. I used them on my grand- father who has Alzheimer's and immediately my family and the nursing home staff has noticed a difference in his behavior.

Another very interesting result of this study was the influence that thoughts have on our frequency as well. Negative thoughts can actually lower someone's frequency by 12 MHZ and positive thoughts can raise someone's frequency by 10 MHZ. Attitude is very important, but didn't we always know that?

Pure, therapeutic essential oils can be used as a compress, inhaled, used in baths, dishwasher, washing machines, dryers, water distillers, filters, cleaning, disinfecting, diffused, taken internally , and used in painting to lessen the fumes.

I hope you include these pure therapeutic essential grade oils in your everyday life, and you choose to buy pure therapeutic grade oils, so you can derive the greatest benefit you can and have optimal health now and in the future.

I'll give the best example I can give of an all purpose essential oil that has been named the most versatile of all oils:

LAVENDER: (Lavandula angustifolia, CT Linalol)

Botanical Family: Labiate(mint)

Extraction method origin: Steam distilled from flowering tip- France, Idaho,Utah

Chemical constituents: Monoterpenes: a and b pinene, camphene;

Sesquiterpenes; Alcohols (45%): linalol, geraniol, borneol, lavendulol;

Esters: linalyl acetate(30-34%), lavenduyl acetate; Oxides: 1,8 cineol;

Ketones; Sesquiterpenones; Aldehydes; Lactones; Coumarins

Properties: Analgesic, Anti-coagulant, Anti-convulsive, anti-depressant, antifungal, antihistamine, anti-inflammatory, antiseptic, antispasmodic, antitoxic, cardiotonic, regenerative, and sedative.

French Medicinal Uses: Acne, Allergies, Burns (cell renewal), Cramps (leg), Dandruff, Diaper Rash, Flatulence, Hair Loss, Herpes, Indigestion, Insomnia,

Lower Blood Pressure, Lymphatic System Drainage, Menopausal conditions, Mouth Abscess, Nausea, Phlebitis, Pre-Menstrual Conditions, Scarring (minimizes), Stretch Marks, Tachycardia, Thrush, Water Retention.

Other Possible Uses: Lavender is a universal oil that has traditionally been known to balance the body and to work wherever there is a need. If in doubt, use Lavender. It may help Arthritis, Asthma, Balancing Body Systems, Boils, Bronchitis, Bruises, Carbuncles, Cold Sores, Convulsions, Depression, Ear aches, Fainting, Gall stones, Hay fever, Headaches, Heart (irregularity) High Blood Pressure, Hives, Hysteria, Insect Bites, Bee stings, Infection, Influenza, Injuries, Laryngitis, Migraine Headaches, Mouth Abscess, Reduce Mucous, Nervous Tension, Pineal Gland (activates), Respiratory Function, Rheumatism, Skin Conditions (eczema, psoriasis, rashes), Sprains, Stress, Sunburns (including lips), Sunstroke, Tension, Throat Infections, Tuberculosis, Typhoid Fever, Whooping Cough, and Wounds.

Body systems affected: Cardiovascular System, Emotional Balance, Nervous system, Skin.

Aromatic Influence: It promotes Consciousness, Health, Love, Peace, and general sense of Well Being.

Application: Apply to Vita Flex Points and directly on area of concern; diffuse.

Blend Classification: Enhancer and Modifier and Equalizer

Blends with: Most oils especially citrus oils, chamomile, clary sage, and geranium.

Frequency: Emotional and Spiritual; approximately 118.

CHAPTER SEVEN.
COLON HYDROTHERAPY AND
LIVER DETOXIFICATION:

This is the most important subject of this book. YOU CANNOT HAVE OPTIMAL HEALTH WITHOUT A REGULAR PROGRAM OF INTERNAL CLEANSING. Important to note: REGULAR CLEANSING PROGRAM. I've actually spoken to people who have tried colon irrigation or colon hydrotherapy once or twice and said I really didn't notice a difference. Well it's taken years of creating a toxic environment and it will take years to reverse the damage that you've done to it. We have to take self responsibility for our sick bodies, stop making excuses, and actually be consistent about our behavioral changes. Then you'll see positive changes over time and be motivated to keep moving ahead. You have to give it a fighting chance, notice I said a FIGHTING chance, not once or twice, but consistent hard work.

Why should I cleanse my body?

With our environment being so polluted whether it's the air we breathe, the water we drink, or the food we eat, the residues are left behind in our bodily tissues. Our imperfect bodies don't have a fighting chance if we don't first cleanse our bodies and then put in clean healthy whole foods in it. What happens if we leave it to chance? Anything from acne to cancer will set in and take hold.

Proof of this is found in samples of hair, blood, urine, body fat, muscle, brain, and even in tumors.

Over time, our liver that performs the task of neutralizing over 5,000 known chemicals , cannot keep up with the overdose of toxins on a daily basis. Then add a typical American diet that is loaded with pesticides, antibiotics, hormones, xenoestrogens, (cheap synthetic estrogens that cause cancer), additives, preservatives, food colorings, excitotoxins, artificial ingredients, and pharmaceutical drugs, your poor liver is exhausted and always running behind. No wonder we are exhausted, crabby, and unmotivated. Our bodies are POLLUTED, AND NEEDS HEALING. Healing cannot begin without first internal cleansing. You can eat a raw diet, drink a gallon of water a day, and exercise and still not be healthy. I myself have done only this, as well as plenty of other people, without internal cleansing and has had minimal results. IF your body is internally coated with candida, pesticides, and other toxic substances, your body will not get the adequate nutrition it needs to perform everyday functions let alone allow you to feel vital.

Dr. Heather Taylor-Hewett, N.D., C.H.P., C.C.H.

How do I get started?

I suggest starting with cleansing your sewage system made up of your colon, liver, and kidneys. Colon cancer is the number one killing cancer right now. If only the medical profession would just recommend to their patients colon hydrotherapy and regular colon cleansing.How many lives would be saved each year? You can start on a colon cleanse program, by taking an herbal Colon Cleanse capsule that cleans and strengthens the digestive tract. The herbs used in the product stimulates the peristaltic action (intestinal muscular movement) of the colon and over time may strengthen the muscles of the large intestines. It also may help to disinfect, soothe, and heal the mucous membrane lining of the entire digestive system. It also aids in digestion, relieves gas, cramps, and cleanses the gallbladder and bile ducts, assisting in the elimination of candida albicans and parasites. (I recommend American Botanicals products for herbal cleansing products.) I recommend a raw food diet, while doing a 2- week colon cleanse program. Next, colon hydrotherapy is recommended, normally a series of six is advisable. Some people need more, of course, no two colons are alike. During the colon hydrotherapy treatments, I strongly advise taking the colon cleanse products; intestinal formula number 1and formula number 2. The treatments will be more effective when these cleansers are used in conjunction. Intestinal formula number 2 is a strong purifier and intestinal vacuum. It works like a clay mask that you would use on your face. It works as a vacuum pulling out old unwanted matter, leaving behind clean toned skin. The number 2 formula draws out old fecal matter from the walls of the colon and bowel pockets. It also aids in the removal of poisons, toxins, parasites, and heavy metals such as mercury and lead. Next, after your colon is relatively clean,(I say this because, it took years of toxic sludge to build up, it may take a year or two depending on your previous lifestyle and age to completely clean out your colon) you need to do a parasite clean up of your entire body. The intestinal formulas take care of the colon but you can have parasites hiding out anywhere in your body. Your liver, muscles, stomach, small intestine, heart, brain, literally anywhere. Parasites are very hard to kill. You need to use something strong and pure at the same time. I only recommend "*Young Living Essential Oils*" I've used many other oils and anti-parasitic cleanses and not been nearly as successful as I have been now. I would not cheaply try to promote a product, I'm not being paid to endorse their products. I have seen miracles happen with these oils. Beware of cheap inferior oils they don't work the same! I recommend *Di-Tone*, *Nutmeg*, *Lemon*, *Clove*, *Anise, fennel, Hyssop, Melaleuca*, *Mountain savory*, *Mugwort, Oregano*, *Tangerine*, *Tarragon,* and *Thyme*. After the parasite cleanse I recommend a kidney, then a liver flush. I recommend using American Botanicals kidney and liver teas and tinctures for a basic cleanse. Five days on each ,and then follow the directions on the packages and bottles. You need to do at least a modified fast on the cleanse. The liver won't dump toxins efficiently if you're not doing a fast.

You don't want to eat too much fat on the cleanse or any type of refined sugar, junk food , meat, dairy, or anything that isn't raw. The purpose of that is so you won't tax the liver. Detoxing is a taxing experience for the body and liver. You can also try JUVATONE and JUVACLEANSE by *Young Living Essential oils*. They cleanse the liver wonderfully and also chelates heavy metals out of the body. I have had great success with my patients and myself with these products. My urine and hair mineral analysis showed a mercury level of 17% before I started using Juvacleanse and after my tests came back at 2% just in one month time period after using these products. I was going to do Intravenous chelation, but after finding out it causes vascular damage I decided to investigate other options. I've had great success with these products across the board.

Why is cleaning my liver so important to optimal health?

Here are the facts:

- Your liver is your first line of defense against all invaders.

- It is the most metabolically complex organ in the entire human body.

- Produces bile to help absorb fats and fat soluble vitamins

- Removes or neutralizes poisons from the blood

- Produces immune cells to stop infection

- Removes germs and bacteria from the blood

- Makes proteins that regulate blood clotting

- It filters and processes all food, nutrients, alcohol, drugs, and other materials that enter the bloodstream and letting them pass, breaking them down or storing them.

- Makes and breaks down many hormones, including cholesterol, testosterone and estrogen

- Regulates blood sugar levels

The quality of virtually every function our body performs depends on our liver. Our liver is also the anchor of all emotions. All negative emotions we experience are stored there.

Yes, the liver is an integral part of vital health. We must treat it with tender loving care. We do this by controlling what we eat and drink. We can't completely control our environment 100% of the time, but we can control what we put in our mouth.

Liver Stressors We Can Avoid:

- Toxins such as, pharmaceutical drugs, parasites, pesticides, petrochemicals, ANY AND ALL PHARMACEUTICAL DRUGS!

- Poor diet

- Too much iron

- Alcohol and recreational drugs

Even medical doctors say that before most diseases develop, the liver was malfunctioning and not doing its job. Oncologists even have said that long before a person develops cancer, almost always the liver was weak and not protecting the patient. REMEMBER THE MAIN FUNCTION OF THE LIVER IS TO PROTECT US FROM THE FORMATION OF DISEASE. So it stands to reason if we have anything from acne to high cholesterol to cancer we need to cleanse and detoxify the liver. The liver also has hundreds even thousands, of cholesterol formations in the shape of stones as well . The gallbladder isn't the only place where stones reside. If you have stones in your gallbladder you have stones in your liver. A great liver flush I put my patients as well as myself on is <u>Dr Hulda Clark's flush</u>. This flush consists of a ½ cup of Organic cold pressed olive oil, 4 tablespoons of epsom salts, and fresh organic lemon or grapefruits. The exact instructions can be found at <u>www.curezone.com</u>. Click on " liver cleanse," then read the explanation of the liver and gallbladder cleanse then follow the directions carefully in order to achieve optimal results. I'm not publishing the directions because I want you to start a colon and parasite cleanse program first. If you don't do this, you will get seriously ill. So please follow my protocol first before starting any liver and gallbladder flush program.

How often should these cleanses be done?

The colon cleanse program should be an ongoing program. The parasite, liver, gallbladder, kidney flush should be done every 3 months. If you have a serious problem or illness, the liver -gallbladder flush can be done every 2 weeks until your problem clears up then you can go into the maintenance phase. I strongly recommend having colon hydrotherapy done <u>during</u> and <u>after </u>a liver flush with a <u>coffee additve</u>. The organic coffee causes the liver to purge toxins.

As I say to my patients happy flushing!

CHAPTER EIGHT.
POISONS THAT WILL
SABOTAGE ANYONE'S HEALTH
AND WELL BEING

Pharmaceutical drugs- They are a menace to society in many ways. At best, they're a quick- fix, a band aid. At their worst, they're causing mania, mass hysteria, and suicides. My biggest concern is the amount of antidepressants, mood stabilizers, and MAOIs that are being prescribed. I've fought depression since I was 13 years old myself, and when it was suggested to me to try antidepressants, I was 22 years old. I was assured that they were safe and that I was chemically imbalanced. Of course I believed them, they were the doctors. I immediately started experiencing horrific side effects that weren't even listed. I called the doctor in a panic and she said it was something else that I was doing because no one had reported those side effects. I knew my body better than anyone, and I figured it to be the antidepressants. At the time, I was on Xanex and Serzone. Over the years, I had complained and they just put me on something else. They seem to work for about a month and then I would crash into suicidal depression, abusing food and alcohol. I went into a self- destruction mode. By the time I was 24, I hired the best therapists, psychiatrists, and nutritionist. I was told I had everything from unipolar depression to manic depression (bi-polar) to schizoaffective disorder. They scared me into staying on several medications at once. I look back and I'm shocked that I was able to drive and function on those drugs and dosages. Until one day, I was with a friend and I was walking upstairs and blacked out, fell backwards and was unconscious. A friend did C.P.R. and revived me while the ambulance was called and on its way. I remember waking up in the hospital and hearing the staff asking me whether I had been raped because my face looked like it had been badly beaten. That woke me up once and for all with the drugs I was on. What if I had been walking upstairs with my 18 month old at the time? So I decided that was it, I'm firing my so- called "experts" on depression, and going off these drugs cold-turkey once and for all. So I picked the next weekend and laid in bed for three days and shook, vomited, and hallucinated like an addict coming off of street drugs. I knew just from that it was all a lie that antidepressants and mood stabilizers weren't addictive. That was exactly one year and six months ago. I've never felt better in my life. I just didn't come off without employing a new lifestyle, including nutritional, neurotransmitter, and detoxification support. I also am not suggesting going off cold turkey without the help of a certified naturopathic doctor. Please don't go to a psychiatrist, for they will just advise you to stay on the medication. Make use of alternative medicine avenues so you can make the healthiest break from the medicines as possible. A book I recommend is Prozac from Panacea to pandora this is a must read about the aftermath of antidepressants and any and all psychotropic drugs and the implications of being on them even temporarily. The author Dr. Ann Blake Tracy, is the leading expert on psychotropic drugs. She' s always called in on high profile cases regarding trials where people committed crimes (mainly murder) while under the influence of psychotropic drugs. I say under the influence because these drugs are mind- altering and are not to be trusted. Please visit www.drugawareness.com. You can find the F.D.A.'s decision to order these pharmaceutical companies to amend their commercials from not saying their drugs are non addictive. They **are** addictive and mind altering and has ruined the lives of many families. Please reconsider the alternatives   a healthy diet consisting of: raw foods, essential oils, detoxification, and neurotransmitter support. Please do not do this on your own, see an alternative medicine doctor.

- I already spoke earlier of excitoxins. Stay away from these additives, they cause brain damage.

- Chlorinated water is another poison that is not spoken of often. Chlorine is one the most toxic and reactive elements known to man. Yes it is put in the public water supply and it creates disinfection; byproducts that can cause cancer, birth defects, and miscarriage. It also inhibits thyroid function, interfering with its uptake of iodine and the amino acid, tyrosine and, therefore, slowing down metabolism, circulation, and immune function. You may say I don't swim in chlorinated pools and I drink distilled water. If you take a shower or bath without a antichlorine filter you are inhaling chlorine through your nose and lungs. This is an even more dangerous method of exposure because it enters your brain and bloodstream a more effective rate. So get a filter immediately!

- Food additives, Pesticides, Preservatives, Antibiotics used in foods. (They are highly carcinogenic and contain xenoestrogens). They tax your immune system.

- Xenoestrogens -(synthetic estrogens) these estrogens lead to estrogen dominance and are implicated in many forms of cancer, endemetriosis, fibroid tumors, cystic breasts, just to name a few. They interfere with the thyroid hormone which interferes with your emotional and physical metabolism. They are found in shampoos, lotions, perfumes, hairspray, cosmetics, cow's milk, soybeans, birth control pill, drugs like premarin (pregnant horse urine) and plastics. This is an important issue to consider; children are being affected as well. For example, girls are starting their periods way too soon. The average age is now 13 for a girl to start her period when it should be around 16 years of age. Stay away from these synthetic estrogens.

- Mercury amalgam or silver fillings- they contain 50% mercury and are highly toxic. When you chew, brush your teeth, or drink hot liquid , your fillings are releasing vapors that are highly toxic. According to the World Health Organization Environmental Health criteria 118 document on inorganic mercury.

The "WHO" document clearly states that the largest estimated average daily intake and retention of mercury and mercury compounds in the general population, not occupationally exposed, is from dental almagams, not from food or air. Silver fillings cause mouth-oral cavity: bleeding gingiva, metallic taste, burning tongue. It affects the central nervous system by affecting concentration difficulties, impaired memory, sleep disturbances, lack of initiative, nervousness. It also affects the gastrointestinal tract.

- Alcohol and recreational drugs- They possess many carcinogenic compounds and alcohol contains xenoestrogens.

- Refined sugar- implicated in heart disease by causing high cholesterol, diabetes, hyperglycemia, hypoglycemia, tears down the nervous system, and wreaks havoc on the immune system. A little for some people is o.k. but not everyone is able to handle refined sugar. Stevia is a great alternative as well as "*grade b*" organic maple syrup. Sugar also contributes to bone mineral loss by causing an acid environment in the body. Try to only consume, if you must, maybe 20 grams a day.

There are poisonous substances to stay away from that I will list; emphasizing the importance in reading all labels (even while shopping at a health food store).These chemicals are found in products such as ; shampoos, cleaning products, deodorants, soaps, clothes, dry cleaning, tap water, cosmetics, etc.

These chemicals are carcinogenic and is implicated in causing nervous system , cancer, skin irritations, and other diseases:

Dr. Heather Taylor-Hewett, N.D., C.H.P., C.C.H.

Acetone

Alcohol

Alpha-Terpineol

Aluminum

Ammonium Compounds

Azo Colors, Azo Compounds

Benzophenone

Benzyl Acetate

Benzyl Alcohol

Butylated Hydroxyanisole (BHA)

Camphor

Carbomer 934 & 40

Cetyl alcohol

Cetyl Lactate, Myristate, Palmitate, Stearate

Chloroform

Cocamide DEA

Collagen

diethanolamine (DEA)

D&S Colors

Dihydroxyacetone (DHA)

EDTA (Ethylenedinitrilo)

Ethyl acetate (on EPA's hazardous waste list)

Fluoride

Flourocarbons

Formaldehyde

Glycerin

Glycols

Imidazolidinyl Urea

Isopropyl Palmitate & Lanole

Lauramide DEA

Limonene

Linalool

Methyl, Propyl and Butyl Paraben

Mineral oil (manufactured from crude oil)

Oleyl Betaine

PEG (polythylene Glycol)

Pentane

Petrolatum

Propyl Gallate

Propylene Glycol (antifreeze)

Propylene Glycol Stearate

PVP

Dr. Heather Taylor-Hewett, N.D., C.H.P., C.C.H.

PVP

Sodium C 14- 16 & Olefin Sulfonate

Sodium Cetyl Sulfacte

Sodium Laurel Sulfate

Sodium Laureth Sulfate (SLES)(engine degreaser)

Sorbitan Stearate

Stearalkonium Chloride

Synthetic Fragrances

Talc

Triethanolamine (TEA) Diethanolamine (DEA)

Many of the "hyped" ingredients - procollagen, collagen, elastin, cross-linked elastin, and hylauronic acids found in most cosmetic brands cannot penetrate the skin because of high molecular weight and are of little benefit. Other virtually useless ingredients are insoluble, oil based vitamin A (Retinyl Palmitate), Placental extracts, and Royal Bee Jelly.

There are actually 880 chemicals in everyday products known to be carcinogenic, harmful, toxic, or cause birth defects. I was once told by a chemist,(who worked for a large artificial nail company) that you would have to bathe in these chemicals everyday in order for us to be affected to the degree of getting a disease. Well, guess what? We do bathe ourselves by means of the environment, food and water. We get multiple exposures daily to these chemicals, and in the meantime, these chemicals bio-accumulate (build up in fatty tissues, organs such as brain, liver, kidneys, and lungs). Unfortunately, cancer or other chronic disease doesn't appear immediately; it can take up to 5-20 years for disease to appear and hormone disrupters don't often show up until the next generation, but they do affect our children.

- Vaccines- all vaccines are immune suppressing; that is, they depress our immune functions. The chemicals in vaccines depress our immune system. The virus present depresses immune function, and the foreign DNA/RNA from animal tissues depresses immunity. When our immune system is depressed we're vulnerable to all pathogens and disease.

Vaccinations reduce our immunity in many important ways:

1) Vaccines contain many chemicals and heavy metals, like mercury and aluminum, which are in themselves immuno-suppressing. Mercury actually causes changes in the lymphocyte activity and decreases lymphocyte viability.

2) Vaccines contain foreign tissues and foreign DNA/ RNA which act to suppress the immune system via graft-vs-host rejection phenomena.

3) Vaccines alter the metabolic activity of PMNs and reduce their chemotaxic abilities. PMNs are our body's defenses against pathogenic bacteria and viruses.

4) Vaccines suppress our immunity merely by over taxing our immune system, with foreign material such as heavy metals, pathogens and viruses.

5) Vaccines clog our lymphatic system and lymph nodes with large protein molecules that have not been adequately broken down by our digestive processes, since vaccines bypass digestion with injections. This is why vaccines are linked to allergies; they contain large proteins which as circulating immune complexes (CICS) or "klinkers" which cause our body to become allergic.

6) Vaccines deplete our body of vital immune enhancing nutrients, such as vitamin C, A, and zinc, which are needed for a strong immune system. It is nutrients like these that primes our immune system, feeds the white blood cells and macrophages and allows them to function optimally.

7) Vaccines are neurotoxic and slow the level of nervous transmission, communications to the brain and other tissues. Now we know that some lymphocytes communicate directly with the brain through a complex set of neurotransmitters. Altering these factors will depress our immunity.

True immunity comes from good nutrition. Vaccines are being found to contribute to Autism, AIDS, Cancer, Allergies, and other Autoimmune system disorders. Seriously, reconsider vaccinating your children. Yes, there are laws concerning children being vaccinated, but thanks to our Constitutional rights, you can get a doctor's note supporting your stand. Check your local laws and find an alternative medicine doctor that can help you with this issue.

Believe me, I could be all day listing known poisons we come in contact with everyday but these are the most common forms. The list will need to be updated on a daily basis. Check the internet regularly, to keep yourself informed of poisons that will sabotage anyone's health.

Good health to you!

REFERENCES:

Alternative Medicine -The definitive Guide by Burton Goldberg

Detox For Life by Loree Taylor Jordan

Detoxification by Linda Page, N.D, P.h.d..

Essential Oils Desk Reference by Essential Science Publishing

Excitoxins- The Taste That Kills by George R. Schwartz, M.D.

Fast Food Nation by Eric Schlosser

Herbal Antibiotics by Stephen Harrod Buhner

Homeopathy Made Simple by Phillip L. Bournet M.D.

The Metabolic Typing Diet by William Wolcott and Trish Fahey

The No Grain Diet by Dr. Joseph Mercola with Alison Levy

Reference Guide For Essential Oils by Connie and Alan Higley

ABOUT THE AUTHOR

Dr. Heather Taylor-Hewett was moved to become a Naturopathic Doctor after she had great success in treating her own illnesses, as well as her oldest son. She had undergone many frustrating experiences, to say the least, with conventional Medicine. After many disappointments with conventional Medicine treatments, she was prompted to try alternative medicine. After having much success, she decided to get in this integrative field of medicine as soon as possible. She attended Blair College of Natural Health and worked hard to receive certification in Clinical Nutrition and Herbal Medicine. She then went on to receive a Doctorate in Naturopathy. Dr. Taylor-Hewett sees patients on a regular basis, and is passionate about helping people heal themselves with professional help.

www.ingramcontent.com/pod-product-compliance
Lightning Source LLC
Chambersburg PA
CBHW020349290526
45785CB00005B/2198